SUGAR

WHAT YOU NEED TO KNOW
ABOUT SUGAR CONSUMPTION

ALI MOHAMMED

ISBN: 9798353522768

DEDICATION

My appreciation goes to Almighty God for making this book a success. Without Him, I wouldn't have been able to come this far. My mother (Fatima) owns the credit for giving birth to a responsible boy and to everyone who contributed for this book to have seen the light of the day, I say thank you.

CONTENTS

Table of Contents

INTRODUCTION

Sugar is poison. High fructose corn syrup causes cancer. Putting sarcasm aside, too much sugar is a bad idea and high fructose corn syrup (HFCS) isn't better. But neither is inherently good or evil. Despite what the media may say, a little added sugar isn't going to instantly kill anyone.

Added sugars make things sweeter and tastier. They have a number of positive qualities when baking and bring a smile to both young and old. Sugar tastes so good that most American adults can credit 14.6% of their daily calories from added sugars.

While sugar may make our taste buds happy, it isn't very nutritious. It contains energy but not much else. It is essentially "empty calories" meaning that you get no nutritional benefit, aside from instant blood-sugar spiking energy, from consuming it.

Sugar comes in many different forms in food. Most healthy foods, including fruits, vegetables, dairy, and grains, contain naturally occurring sugars or carbohydrates. Processed foods can contain naturally occurring carbohydrates plus added sugars. These added sugars come in many forms, and some are labeled "natural" to be more appealing to consumers.

The FDA does not have a definition of the word natural; they do allow the word to be used if a product has no added colors, artificial flavors or synthetic substances but this is a loose regulation. "Naturally" added sugars like agave nectar, honey and maple syrup also have calories but are reported to have more helpful nutrients as well, like B vitamins, selenium and iron. Unfortunately, in order to see those nutritional benefits, you'd have to eat quite a bit of these added sugars each day.

Processed foods, like boxed, canned, wrapped or frozen (not usually fruits and vegetables), generally contain added sugars, though not all do. Processed foods must go through processing (obviously) which tends to remove essential nutrients. Generally speaking, the more processed a food is the less nutritious it will be. If a food is processed, look at the label and ingredients to figure out what it contains and whether you should be consuming it. According to the American Heart Association; added sugar, in all forms, should be restricted to no more than 6 teaspoons (24 grams) a day for women (approximately 100 calories) and 9 teaspoons a day for men (approximately 150 calories) or less than 5% of total daily calories. For label reference 4 grams of sugar=1 teaspoon of sugar and 1 gram of sugar=4 calories.

TYPES OF SUGAR

You may say that you cannot live without sugar but you will be surprise that not everyone knows how sugar could be available in their table or in their coffee every morning. As mentioned above, sugar could be found in almost every plant you could find on earth but commercially, sugar is extracted from sugarcane or sugar beet. Sugar is the English word but the etymology comes from Arabic _sukkar_. As you may have known there are a lot of types of sugar and some of them are mostly found in every home as the list below:

1. Granulated sugar is the most common type of sugar that usually available in your table to be mixed with tea or coffee and added to foods.
2. Brown sugar is mostly used in baking because it gives more texture and color.
3. Powder sugar is actually used in baking as well especially types of baking that required sugar to be quickly dissolved.
4. Sugar cubes are available in two types, white and brown. Sugar cubes actually made from granulated sugar or brown sugar which are pressed in block shape and usually serve with coffee or tea.
5. Liquid sugar is just another type of granulated sugar that is dissolved in water.

Those are only some types of sugar that you commonly find around you. Those are mostly already refined because they have through several process that affect its purity until they arrive in your table.

10 HEALTH BENEFITS OF SUGAR

Sugar earns its bad reputation because it is always associated with the main factor that causes the spike of blood sugar level in diabetic patients, obesity and tooth decay. However, do you know that no human could live without sugar? Even your tongue knows better that everything sweet always win over others flavors. It is because there are a lot of benefits of sugar for health, so no one will survive without consuming sugar. The main compound of sugar is glucose and even in the tartest fruit you could find on earth may contain glucose. In other words, there is no way you could avoid sugar unless you eat nothing.

- **Sugar Is Excellent Calories Source:** Calories are always associated with weight gain and obesity. That's why a lot of people are spending most of their times counting calories they consume. However, calories are the reasons why you have energy to do some activities, that's why whenever you consume calories is better to find a way to burn it.

- **Sugar for Insulin Benefits**: Insulin is essential to the production of energy. Without which, glucose will remain in your bloodstream and cause the spike of blood sugar. Insulin will turn glucose into energy that you could use to do all the activities all day.

- **Sugar is Excellent Energy Source**: If you need immediate energy booster, sugar is the excellent source. That's why, when you add sugar to your coffee in the morning, the combination of caffeine and sugar will give you the energy booster you really need. However, you need to careful because too much sugar will give you too much energy but only for a while, so you should spend the rest of the day being sluggish and unfocused.

- **Sugar to Store Energy**: Sugar has prominent role in human body metabolism because glucose found in sugar if it is not used or turned into energy will be stocked in your body cells as glycogen. This compound is excellent source of energy wherever you need it. However, too much stored glycogen in your body cells will be turned into fat that will lead to conditions like weight gain and obesity.

- **Sugar is Solution to Instant Mood Booster**: Whenever you feel sad or moody, try to eat candy or add more sugar to your herbal tea. It is because sugar contains some compound that will send certain signal to your brain to produce more dopamine, a hormone that is responsible to euphoric feeling. It will improve your mood and make you a little happier.

- **Sugar Contains Glycolic Acid**: If you are not familiar with glycolic acid; it is type of acid compound that responsible to protect your skin from sun-damaged and premature aging and sugar is the natural source of this glycolic acid. However, since covering your skin with sugar is not the solution to protect it from bad effects of UV rays, using sunscreen is still highly recommended while sugar is only used for regular treatment.

- **Sugar for Natural Skin Scrub**: How much money you should spend to go to spa or purchasing expensive skin scrub products? Well, you could save more money if you know how to make homemade and natural skin scrub made from sugar. Sugar contains AHA or Alpha Hydroxy Acid which is an excellent exfoliant. It will exfoliate the top layer of your skin to eliminate the dead skin cells and reveal the natural skin glowing.

- **Sugar for Kissable Lips**: Well, just like sugar is effective to remove dead skin cells in your body, sugar is also excellent to remove dead skin cells in your lips. Just by applying the mixture of sugar and honey to your lips every day, you could kiss goodbye peeling and chapped lips for good. Instead, you will get smooth and kissable lips.

- **Sugar to Eliminate Blackheads**: Not only for your body skin and lips, you could also apply sugar as face scrubs. However, since skin face is more sensitive than body skin, you should mix it with some ingredients that give more benefits to your skin face like sesame oil. Applying them to your skin face and then rub it slowly in circle to help removing the blackheads and then wash them off with warm and then cold water to close the open pores after the scrubbing.

- **Sugar to Lighten the Toned Skin Areas**: It is very annoying when your skin products cannot deal with some toned skin areas like in your armpits, elbows and knees. However, you don't need to worry anymore because the same natural skin scrubs you have made for your body could be applied to those tone areas as well for smoother and healthier skin.

So, sugar is probably making your coffee sweet, your mood better and your skin smoother but too much of it will give you nothing but harmful and scary effects. Furthermore, if you really want to avoid sugar, you could avoid all kinds of refined sugar and instead consume the raw or natural sugar only for all the benefits of sugar for health. For sweetener alternative, don't fall to some commercials that said about corn-sugar is better than sugar, well corn-sugar is much worse than the actual sugar. Honey and natural fruit juice are still the best sweetener alternative in this matter.

9 NEGATIVE EFFECTS Of SUGAR

Sugar can give you wrinkles and adds age to your face. Scientists from the Leiden University Medical Centre in the Netherlands measured the blood sugar levels of 600 men and women aged between 50 and 70. They then showed photographs of these people to 60 separate participants and found that those with higher blood sugar looked older than those with lower blood sugar levels.

In fact, for every 1mm/liter increase in blood sugar, the perceived age of that person rose by five months.

1. **Sugar is also associated with acne.** Foods ranked high on the Glycemic Index such as sugar and refined carbs have been associated with greater amounts of acne on the face and body, according to the latest research. A study of Australian men showed that those who ate a diet with a low glycemic load saw a great reduction in overall acne. It was a small study with only 23 men, but it's still food for thought.

2. **Sugary drinks cause an 83% increase in developing type II diabetes.** One study of 91,249 women showed that those who consumed 1 sugar-sweetened beverage a day had an 83% increased risk of developing type II diabetes compared to those who had only 1 a month.

3. **People who eat sugar are at a much higher risk of cancer.** There has been a direct link seen between breast, and colon cancer with sugar consumption. This is likely due to the fact that insulin is one of the key factors behind the growth and multiplication of

cells, and sugar spikes insulin to abnormally high levels.

4. **Sugar can ruin your teeth.** A study by the American journal of clinical nutrition showed that sugar destroys the healthy bacteria in our mouth. This can cause tooth erosions and may dim that bright smile. What about sugar and weight gain?

5. **Sugar is the premier definition of empty calories.** It has no real nutritional value, no nutrients, no minerals, no proteins, and no fiber. Because of this lack of nutrients.

6. **Sugar makes you feel hungry.** In a study by Yale University, those that consumed sugar had an increased appetite and desire from more food. So not only does sugar fill you with empty calories, but it also makes you want more of those calories.

This process happens because sugar screws up hormonal levels in the body, which leads to our next point.

7. **Sugar blocks leptin and raises insulin to supernatural levels.** Leptin is the hormone in charge of telling us we're full and need to stop eating. It also tells us we have energy and should go out and use that energy. Sugar consumption blocks this hormone from doing its job and from reaching the brain.

Sugar also spikes insulin, making it very hard for the body to access and burn the stored fat on our bodies.

8. **Sugar causes belly fat.** Numerous studies have shown direct links from sugar to increased accumulation of belly fat. This is the worst kind of fat, because it's the one associated with all sorts of diseases including the world's number 1 killer-heart disease. Despite knowing all this, it's hard to stop eating sugar because.

9. **Sugar is addictive.** Similar to drugs like cocaine, scientists have now shown that sugar causes a very similar release of dopamine in the brain. Studies on neuroplasticity have shown that drug users have similar behavioral addictions to those addicted to sugar. Point blank: Sugar is addicting and comes without the immediate social repercussions of frequent drug use. That's why it's so hard to stop eating it.

17 FOODS AND DRINKS THAT ARE SURPRISINGLY HIGH IN SUGAR

Here are 17 foods and drinks that may contain more sugar than you'd think.

1. **Low Fat Yogurt:** Yogurt can be highly nutritious. However, not all yogurt is created equal. Like many other low fat products low fat yogurts often contain added sugar to enhance their flavor.

   For example, a single cup (245 grams) of low-fat yogurt can contain over 45 grams of sugar, which is about 11 teaspoons. This is more than the daily limit for men and women in just a single cup.

   Furthermore, low fat yogurt doesn't seem to have the same health benefits as full fat yogurt. When you're choosing yogurt, look for those that contain the least amount of added sugar. Also, choosing one without fruit and adding your own allows you to control its sugar content and increase its nutritional value.

2. **Barbecue (BBQ) Sauce:** Barbecue (BBQ) sauce can make a tasty marinade or dip.

   However, 2 tablespoons (around 28 grams) of sauce can contain around 9 grams of sugar. This is over 2 teaspoons worth. In fact, around 33% of the weight of BBQ sauce may be pure sugar. If you're liberal with your servings, this makes it easy to consume a lot of sugar without meaning. To make sure you aren't getting too much, check the labels and choose the sauce with the least amount of added sugar. Also, remember to watch your portion size.

3. **Ketchup:** Ketchup is one of the most popular condiments worldwide, but — like BBQ sauce — it's often loaded with sugar. Try to be mindful of your portion size when using ketchup, and remember that a single tablespoon of ketchup contains nearly 1 teaspoon of sugar.

4. **Fruit Juice:** Like whole fruit, fruit juice contains some vitamins and minerals.

   However, when choosing a fruit juice, pick one that's labeled 100% fruit juice, as sugar-sweetened versions can come with a large dose of sugar and very little fiber.

   In fact, there can be just as much sugar in sugar-sweetened fruit juice as there is in a sugary drink like Coke. The poor health outcomes that have been linked to sugary soda may likewise be linked to fruit juices with added sugar.

   Choose whole fruit or 100% fruit juice when possible, and minimize your intake of sugar-sweetened fruit juices. Added sugars are often hidden in foods that we don't even consider to be sweet.

5. **Spaghetti sauce:** As spaghetti sauce. All spaghetti sauces will contain some natural sugar given that they're made with tomatoes.

   However, many spaghetti sauces contain added sugar as well. The best way to ensure you aren't getting any unwanted sugar in your pasta sauce is to make your own.

   However, if you need to buy premade spaghetti sauce, check the label and pick one that either doesn't have sugar on the ingredient list or has it listed very close to the bottom. This indicates that it's not a major ingredient.

6. **Sports Drinks:** Sports drinks Sports drinks can often be mistaken as a healthy choice for those who exercise.
   However, sports drinks are designed to hydrate and fuel trained athletes during prolonged, intense periods of exercise. For this reason, they contain high amounts of added sugars that can be quickly absorbed and used for energy.

   In fact, a standard 20-ounce (591-mL) bottle of a sports drink will contain 32.5 grams of added sugar and 161 calories. This is equivalent to 9 teaspoons of sugar. Sports drinks are therefore categorized as sugary drinks. Like soda and sugar-sweetened fruit juice, they've also been linked to obesity and metabolic disease. Unless you're a marathon runner or elite athlete, you should probably just stick to water while exercising. It's by far the best choice for most of us.

7. **Chocolate Milk:** Chocolate milk is milk that has been flavored with cocoa and sweetened with sugar. Milk itself is a very nutritious drink. It's a rich source of nutrients that are great for bone health, including calcium and protein.

   However, despite having all the nutritious qualities of milk, 1 cup (250 grams) of chocolate milk comes with almost 12 extra grams (2.9 teaspoons) of added sugar.

8. **Granola:** Granola is often marketed as a low-fat health food, despite being high in both calories and sugar. The main ingredient in granola is oats. Plain rolled oats are a well-balanced cereal containing carbs, protein, fat, and fiber.

   However, the oats in granola have been combined with nuts and honey or other added sweeteners, which increases the amount of sugar and calories.

   In fact, 100 grams of granola can contain around 400–500 calories and nearly 5–7 teaspoons of sugar. If you like granola, try choosing one with less added sugar or making your own. You can also add it as a topping to fruit or yogurt rather than pouring a whole bowl.

9. **Flavored Coffees:** Flavored coffee is a popular trend, but the number of hidden sugars in these drinks can be staggering. In some coffeehouse chains, a large flavored coffee or coffee drink can contain 45 grams of sugar, if not much more. That's equivalent to about 11 teaspoons of added sugar per serving.

    Considering the strong link between sugary drinks and poor health, it's probably best to stick to coffee without any flavored syrups or added sugar.

10. **Iced Tea:** Iced tea is usually sweetened with sugar or flavored with syrup. It's popular in various forms and flavors around the world, so its sugar content can vary slightly. Most commercially prepared iced teas will contain around 35 grams of sugar per 12-ounce (340-mL) serving. This is about the same as a bottle of Coke. If you like tea, pick regular tea or choose iced tea that doesn't have any sugars added.

11. **Protein bars:** Protein bars are a popular snack. Foods that contain protein have been linked to increased feelings of fullness, which can aid weight loss. This has led people to believe that protein bars are a healthy snack.

    While there are some healthier protein bars on the market, many contain around 20 grams of added sugar, making their nutritional content similar to that of a candy bar.

When choosing a protein bar, read the label and avoid those that are high in sugar. You can also eat a high protein food such as yogurt instead.

12. **Premade soup:** Soup isn't a food that you generally associate with sugar. When it's made with fresh whole ingredients, it's a healthy choice and can be a great way to increase your vegetable consumption without much effort.

The vegetables in soups have naturally occurring sugars, which are fine to eat given that they're usually present in small amounts and alongside lots of other beneficial nutrients.

However, many commercially prepared soups have a lot of added ingredients, including sugar. To check for added sugars in your soup, look at the ingredient list for names such as:

- sucrose

- barley malt

- dextrose

- maltose

- high fructose corn syrup and other syrups

The higher up on the list an ingredient is, the higher its content in the product. Watch out for when manufacturers list small amounts of different sugars, as that's another sign the product could be high in total sugar.

13. **Breakfast cereal:** Cereal is a popular, quick, and easy breakfast food.

However, the cereal you choose could greatly affect your sugar consumption, especially if you eat it every day. Some breakfast cereals, even those marketed to children, have lots of added sugar. Some contain 12 grams, or 3 teaspoons of sugar in a small 34-gram (1.2-ounce) serving. Check the label and try choosing a cereal that's high in fiber and low in added sugar.

Better yet, wake up a few minutes earlier and cook a quick healthy breakfast with a high protein food like eggs, as eating protein for breakfast can help you lose weight.

14. **Cereal bars:** For on-the-go breakfasts, cereal bars can seem like a healthy and convenient choice.

However, like other "health bars," cereal bars are often just candy bars in disguise. Many contain very little fiber or protein and are loaded with added sugar.

15. **Canned fruits:** All fruit contains natural sugars. However, some canned fruit is peeled and preserved in sugary syrup. This processing strips the fruit of its fiber and adds a lot of unnecessary sugar to what should be a healthy snack.

The canning process can also destroy heat-sensitive vitamin C, although most other nutrients are well preserved. Whole, fresh fruit is best. If you want to eat canned fruit, look for one that has been preserved in juice rather than syrup. Juice has a slightly lower sugar content.

16. **Canned baked beans:** Half the amount of sugar found Baked beans are another savory food that's often surprisingly high in sugar. One cup (254 grams) of regular baked beans contains about 5 teaspoons of sugar. If you like baked beans, you can choose low sugar versions. They can contain about in their full sugar counterparts.

17. **Premade smoothies:** Blending fruits with milk or yogurt in the morning to make yourself a smoothie can be a great way to start your day.

However, not all smoothies are healthy. Many commercially produced smoothies come in large sizes and can be sweetened with ingredients like ice cream or syrup. This increases their sugar content.

Some of them contain ridiculously high amounts of calories and sugar, with over 50 grams (13 teaspoons) of sugar in a single 16- or 20-ounce (473- or 591-mL) serving. For a healthy smoothie, check the ingredient content and be mindful of your portion size.

IS SUGAR ADDICTIVE?

Yes, sugar can be as addictive as drugs and alcohol and is very difficult to avoid due to its presence and addition to many food items. Consuming, or even just thinking about it, can stimulate the brain and release dopamine into the system.

Sugar not only tastes good but is also potentially addictive. Consuming or even thinking about caramel can trigger a dopamine release a neurotransmitter that controls pleasure and reward-motivated behavior, into the system. Studies have shown that this substance can be as addictive as drugs and alcohol. However, it is more difficult to avoid caramel as there are thousands of packaged food items in grocery stores today, with about 80 percent of them containing added sugars.

The main problem, however, comes from what people drink and not what they eat. Drinking a single one of any of today's popular beverages is already over the daily recommendation. The average can of soda contains about 40grams of added sugars while bottles have around 42 grams and one Starbucks coffee contains about 47 grams of added sugars.

CAUSES OF SUGAR ADDICTION

Sugar addiction often sets off a chain reaction of cravings to anything with a high concentration of sugar. How do people develop an addiction to sugar? It starts with a fatigued individual needing a source of energy or a carb-rich meal or drinks in many cases. What happens instantaneously after ingesting the carb-stocked food is that the sugar content of the meal releases chemicals called endorphins inside the body, which reacts with other components to boost the individual's energy. Upon realizing the effectiveness of a carb diet or beverage in supplying substantial energy, a person may unconsciously begin to abuse sugar or become involuntarily dependent on caramel for emotional balance, as a cure for irritability, energy, motivation, and other conditions. Over time, the individual loses control over their intake, leading to a fully developed addiction.

SUGAR ADDICTION AND CO-OCCURRING DISORDERS

The obvious sign of sugar addiction is usually behavioral. The compulsion to consume large amounts of high-sugar drinks, beverages, or food is a clear sign of sugar addiction. The individual in question may adopt the indulgence in excess sugar to deal with life problems and experiences. Such a person often repeatedly talks about cravings for either physical or emotional stability. The peculiarity of sugar addiction is that it often presents with co-occurring disorders.

Sugar Addiction and Binge Eating: Binge eating is a problem that is very common among people who are addicted to sugar. Binge eating means consuming a lot of food or snacks in a very short period of time. This is often followed by a feeling of shame, disgust, and dissatisfaction in one's self. Some individuals first develop an emotional imbalance, and due to depression, they binge eat until they become addicted to sugar. This can happen in reverse.

Sugar Addiction and Alcoholism: The consumption of this substance often leads to the stimulation of dopamine receptors in the brain, which is similar to what happens when one abuses alcohol. Alcoholics often have a craving or sugar withdrawal. The sugar preference genes may be passed down to offspring who may be predisposed to any or both compulsions, depending on their lifestyle.

Sugar Addiction and Emotional Eating: Emotional eating and sugar addiction has been known to go hand-in-hand following a stressful day, handling social and emotional pressures, as well as dealing with life's situations. People enduring emotional stress such as bullying, breakup, and other similar issues or dealing with a damaged reputation, and low self-esteem may result in comfort food such as chocolate, ice cream, candy, and others to deal with their problems.

Addiction to caramel can also accompany compulsive gambling or addiction to video games, when one mixes uncontrolled eating with prolonged playing games or slots.

Sugar Addiction and Anxiety: Anxiety is a mental condition that is characterized by unrest and can affect every aspect of a person's body. Anxiety can cause irregularities in appetite. Some people develop eating disorders like anorexia, while some may start to binge eat, leading to sugar addiction and other secondary health issues.

Why does this happen? The stress-related hormone cortisol is released when a person develops anxiety. This hormonal change works differently in people. For some, it leads to a complete lack of appetite, while for others, it boosts their appetite for sugar-based meals and snacks. This inadvertently leads to excess weight gain and worsens anxiety as depletion in sugar levels immediately leads to depression and fatigue.

Sugar Withdrawal and Detox Symptoms: When people quit this substance, physiological changes occur. Within hours the hormonal levels change. The levels of insulin will start to decrease, allowing the body to access stored fats to burn for energy. After a few days, lipid levels start to drop, especially triglycerides. Over a prolonged period, palate changes, and things that used to taste normal later taste unpleasantly sweet, and palate adjust to require a lot less of it to feel satisfied. These are some of the benefits one will experience after quitting this substance but not before going through a withdrawal phase.

HOW TO QUITE SUGAR INTAKE

There are cases where individuals who realize that they have a sweetener problem seek counseling on how to stop eating sugar. The following are simple techniques on how to stop eating sugar.

Don't Quit It Cold Turkey: The human body relies on many elements of food and drinks to run efficiently; sucrose is one of those elements. This is the reason many health professionals do not recommend that a person cuts it completely out of the diet when attempting to detox. Instead, they recommend that one reduces sugars to a more refined amount, possibly just eating a little fruit after a meal, for example.

Gradual Elimination: Most people who are addicted to sugar find that the best and most effective way to detox is gradually cutting back. This way, withdrawal symptoms are far less noticeable, and a person is more likely to keep that positive feeling of doing something that is good for their health. This makes it less likely that one will give up the detox completely.

When it comes to methods of cutting back, there are a few ways of approaching the detox. One method is only withdrawing for one day a week and gradually increasing that by a measure of time every week until one reaches an ideal level of caramel consumption. An alternative method is to add water to drinks. This way, there is a reduction in the amount of sweetener with every drink. One can gradually reduce it more and more, eventually replacing sugary drinks altogether with a healthier option.

Complete Elimination: Cutting sucrose completely out of the diet would not only enhance withdrawal symptoms, but it would also be incredibly unhealthy in the long run. Furthermore, the idea of not having caramel at all can be detrimental to mentality while attempting to detox.

WHAT ARE THE SYMPTOMS OF SUGAR WITHDRAWAL?

Overcoming sugar addiction comes with its withdrawal and detox symptoms, which a person needs to be aware of, as well as knowing when to expect them and how to manage them. When one removes this substance from the diet, the detox is not necessarily the biggest issue, but the idea that it has a drug-like effect on the body. It is a stimulant, and when taken it away, the body has to adjust and adapt accordingly.

These are some of the withdrawal symptoms one can almost definitely expect when detoxing from sucrose.

Cravings: This happens immediately after one goes cold turkey. One will definitely crave sugar as it has silently become a drug of choice. One will crave it and think about it all the time. This is the first sign that the body is dependent on it because as soon as a person removes it from the diet, the body is asking for it back immediately. This is an indication of a major imbalance in the system, which should spur one to stay on course.

Lethargy: A complete lack of energy follows shortly after as a result of the absence of the primary energy source. As early as 24 hours after ceasing its intake, a person starts to feel this lethargy. One feels like being about to get sick, the body feels heavy, the mind feels dull, and one feels a bit listless and emotionless. A person might even feel a little depressed depending on how dependent the body was on sucrose. There will be some disturbance in mood and probably some issues with thinking clearly and communicating. One needs to stay strong and ride this wave out in the course of detox.

Anxiety: Caramel gives us a temporary boost of energy, and it is similar to a high that makes us happy in the short term. Taking away this source makes our brains react in ways that can manifest as anxiety. According to a 2002 study at Princeton University, this anxiety was observed in rats that were subjects of sweetener dependence and withdrawal. Anxiety was manifested in behaviors such as teeth chattering, paw tremors, and head shaking.

Headaches: Perhaps the most common side effect of quitting sweeteners is the sugar withdrawal headache. It is often recommended to consume small amounts of this substance to relieve the headaches, preferably from fruits. If the headaches are severe, then perhaps quitting cold turkey is not the right choice, and one should try a more gradual approach.

HOW TO DEAL WITH SUGAR WITHDRAWAL SYMPTOMS

A person will go through cravings, irritability, fatigue, and mood swings, to name just a few things. But what is the best way to deal with sugar withdrawal and its symptoms?

One suggestion is a dietary supplement known as glutamine. Glutamine helps to combat sugar withdrawal symptoms by providing the body with a replacement for it, getting energy from an alternative base. Another suggestion commonly made is to drink lots of water. This will help to stay hydrated and combat some of the cravings. Since cravings are mostly driven by the brain's need for some form of reward which is harmful to the body, the best options are usually to tackle the problem with physical and mental techniques. Some ways of dealing with sugar withdrawal are:

Going for a Run or Walk: Exercises are known to release chemicals called endorphins, also known as "feel good" hormones in the brain. This is instrumental in switching off the craving. In cases where one cannot go out for a walk, indoor workouts such as push-ups, squats, and others may suffice.

Eat Healthily: Most sweetener addicts eat, not because they are hungry, but because of an addiction to the sucrose content- the brain signaling for a reward through the release of dopamine. Cravings are often difficult to resist; however, a great way to overcome sugar withdrawal symptoms is to eat a healthy premade diet and have a good stock of healthy sugar-free snacks. Eating regular food may not seem as appetizing, but the feeling of fullness may help curb the habit of extra sugary nibbles.

A Hot Bath: People who used this method found it to be

quite effective. The mechanism behind hot showers and cravings is yet uncertain, but anecdotal reports have consistently suggested that a 5 to 10 minutes hot shower may be all you need when you are experiencing sugar withdrawal symptoms.

As much as these methods are effective for sugar withdrawal symptoms, prevention is always better than a cure. Keeping up a healthy eating habit and exercising often has been found to be the most effective.

Other Ways to Tackle Sugar Withdrawal Symptoms are:

- Eat lots of protein
- Eat plenty of fruits
- Avoid artificial sweeteners
- Always stay hydrated
- Get lots of sleep
- Avoid going long hours without eating
- Stay away from triggers

CONCLUSION

Generally, the best way to combat sugar withdrawal symptoms seems to be to keep the blood sugar levels stable. Replacements for it, such as almond butter or coconut oil, will ensure that one does not suffer a sudden crash in blood sugar levels if one takes a dosage of them every few hours. Alongside the almond butter, a person should maintain a good sleeping and eating pattern. It is also recommended that one does not totally abstain from fruit. Despite its content of natural sugars, the fruit is a vital dietary requirement, and therefore it should still be eaten in moderation. This will help the body to re-adjust to a usual diet and meaning the detox is done as soon as possible in the best possible quality. At the end of it all, sugar is good for you but do not take more than it is required.

ABOUT THE AUTHOR

I am a native of Tolon in the Northern Region of Ghana. I was born in to the family of Mr. and Mrs. Mohammed on the 27th day of March, 1996. I've completed both my elementary and middle school at Tolon and afterwards I had admission in to Yendi Senior High School where I've completed in May 2015 and yet to continue my education.